Thank You

I would like to thank Brandon, Liam, Mom, Dad, and Brittney. Your love and support means the world to me.

THE SIMPLE GUIDE TO

POSTNATAL CARE

FOR FIRST TIME MOMS

BY JASMINE ALLEN

Table of Contents

Introduction

My pregnancy was emotionally difficult. My puritanical well-intentioned mother made it seem like pregnancy was the worst thing that could happen to me from puberty until I was married. My unfulfilled dreams, and the state of my marriage wore on me. I resented the pressure I felt to keep my son. I felt all alone. But my baby was there, and he was a comfort. I loved him. Nesting gave me the courage to tell people that they had two options: get it together, or stay away from me.

My health care experience was terrifying. Beyond the nonsensical treatment for gestational diabetes I received and fear of postpartum depression, my doctor almost caused me to fall from the doctor's office bed in my third trimester. I was demeaned for failed breastfeeding attempts and told to walk on my swollen water retention feet. The nurses didn't even tell me how to use the bathroom.

During my postpartum recovery journey, I figured out a lot of things with the help of my husband, my beautiful baby boy, friend, and a bunch of research. I have decided to use this knowledge to help you in your mommy hood transition, hoping it will be smoother than mine was. I am sharing everything I learned about postpartum self-care including mental health, pelvic floor treatment, and closing diastasis recti.

This book is succinct. If you are anything like me when I was pregnant, you have limited patience. Every time I attempted to read more than five pages, my mind muttered, "F#%$ is all these words."

XOXO,
Jasmine

Essentials

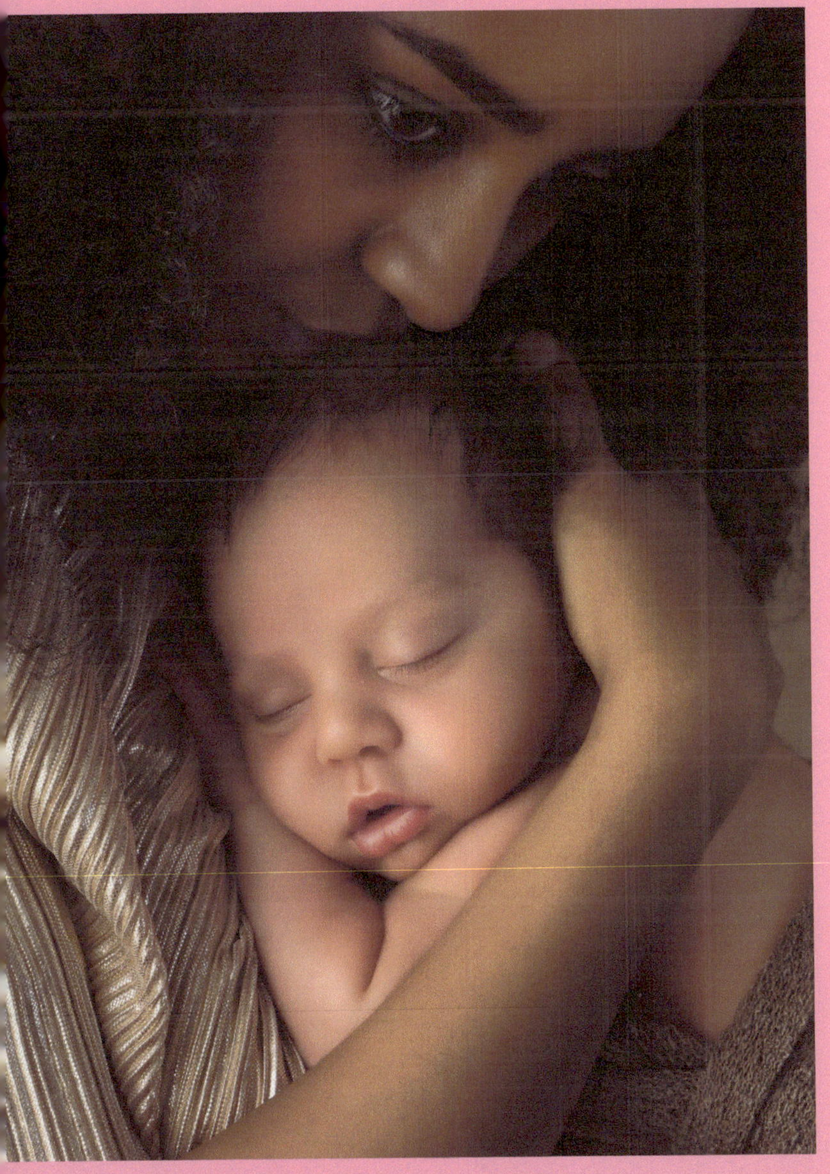

Sleep

So, you have just had a baby, you strong, beautiful, warrior, goddess! Now sit down and rest. Design a sleep schedule. It helps to ask a night owl to stay up until 2AM or 4AM to support the baby and you can wake up at 2PM or 4PM to take care of your baby. If you sleep from 8PM until 4AM or 6PM until 2AM, you will get a full 8 hours of sleep. If you are breastfeeding, you can pump in advance so that another person is prepared for feedings.

Padsickles

Brittney: Girl, you need to make some padsickles.
Me: What are padsickles?

You can pour witch hazel and aloe vera on pads, wrap them back up in the wrapper, and freeze them so that when you are discharged from the hospital, you can relieve vaginal pain by placing cold pads in your underwear.

Icepacks

You can fill ice packs with water, freeze them and rest them on your vagina.

Pro Tip: if you add rubbing alcohol to the pack and freeze it, it will be colder and not melt because alcohol freezes at a lower temperature.

Using the Bathroom

Rinsing your vagina with water during urination is necessary to avoid pain. Spraying Desitin on it can relieve pain after urination.

Hemorrhoids

Doctor: It's just a little hemorrhoid.
Me (when I touch it): A small forest animal must have bit me! Small? These things are huge!

If you want your butt to heal, try Preparation H wipes and gel. You can wipe yourself with Preparation H wipes. Use baby wipes to clean the nozzle of the ointment before inserting it and applying it to your hemorrhoids.

Sitz Bath

Sitz baths are used to relieve genital pain and itching. Sitz bath kits that can be placed on the toilet are ideal because taking a regular bath in a tub could expose you to bacterial infections. Herbal sitz bath remedy mixtures may also be added to help heal your vagina and hemorrhoids.

Breastfeeding

Breastfeeding can be painful. Try to have a happy and optimistic mindset so that you don't grow discouraged or stressed from all the pressure to breastfeed. Identify someone who can be emotionally supportive to you in the process without pushing you to breastfeed, or encouraging you to give up. They may all have good intentions, but it is most helpful if someone understands that you may get frustrated and change your mind. You want the help of someone who can follow your lead.

Sometimes, it takes a few days for your milk to come in. Don't feel defeated if you want to breastfeed, and are having difficulty. Request formula for your child until your milk comes in.

Nipple guards can be used to accommodate breastfeeding for those with flat or inverted nipples and can reduce the physical pressure on your nipple. Nipple covers are useful to prevent leaks on your clothes. You can use nipple cream to treat soreness.

Use a pillow to elevate the baby so you can breastfeed without hurting your back. Good posture prevents unnecessary soreness. Also, relieve the pain of engorged breasts with a warm compress.

Belly Band

Belly bands offer back support as you regain your core strength. It is not necessary to wear it when sitting or sleeping.

Hydration

Drink plenty of water. Staying hydrated supports muscle recovery.

Feet

Stay off your feet and elevate your legs. When I gave birth, my feet were swollen. My nurses told me that walking would relieve the swelling. Wrong! Maybe I should have known better, but that's not the point. My feet had gotten much worse. They were like huge tender balloons. In order to relieve the swelling, you must lift your feet above your hips. It helps to put your feet up on two pillows or adjust the hospital bed for a similar effect. I found shower shoes to be helpful. Shoes, in general, were good because my balance was terrible.

Mental Health

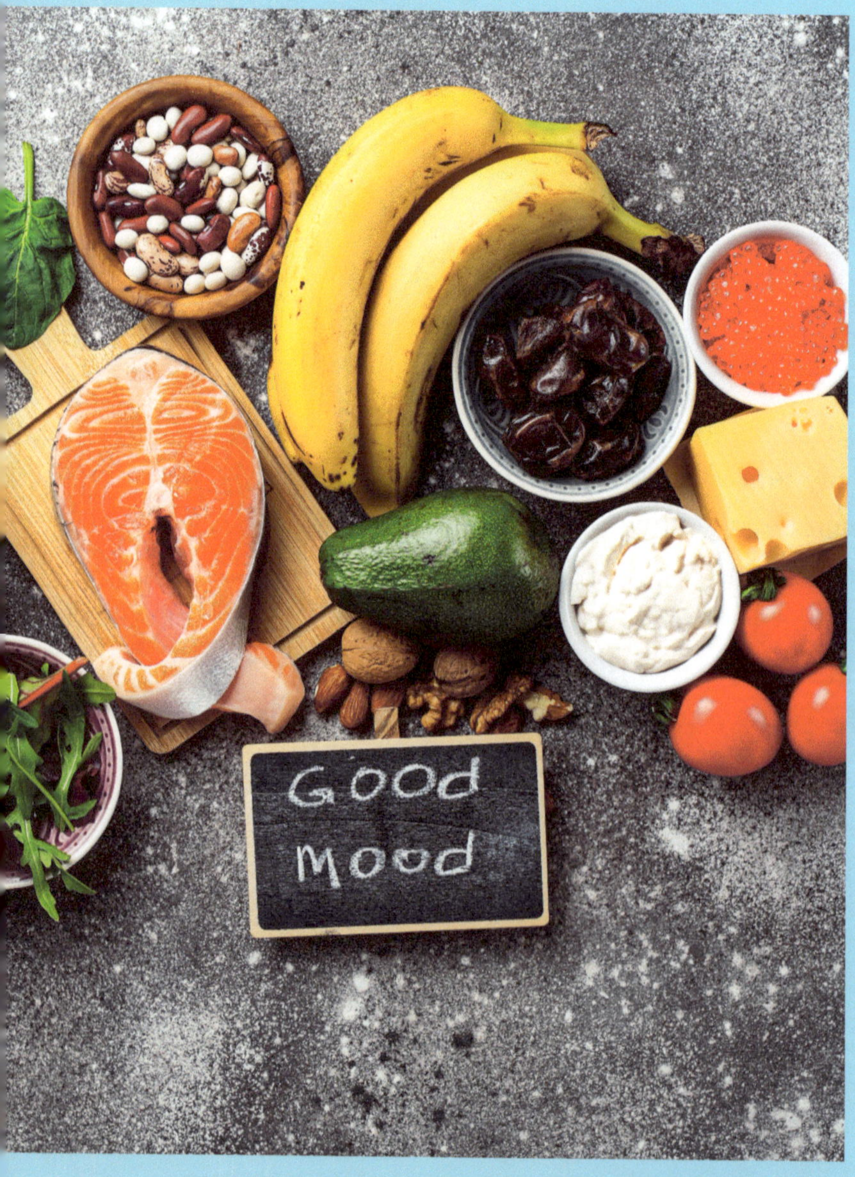

Postpartum Depression

I feared postpartum depression because I have a history of depression. My doctor suggested medication. I didn't want my hair to fall out from using the medication, only to find myself still struggling with depression when my hormones inevitably shifted if I discontinued use. So, I did my own research. I planned to pursue therapy if depression warranted it. I learned how serotonin can boost mood naturally. I considered supplements and the Mediterranean Diet.

The Mediterranean Diet promotes healing and serotonin. The main components of the Mediterranean diet include daily consumption of vegetables, fruits, whole grains and healthy fats; weekly intake of fish, poultry, beans and eggs; moderate portions of dairy products; and limited intake of red meat. I asked my doctor about my dieting plans, and she said that it would be fine. Consult your doctor about your diet plans. I paid close attention to my mood and adjusted my diet when necessary. I also used lavender oil and lavender scented soap to improve my mood.

My personal theory is that some depression is perpetuated by other people disregarding the needs of mothers in a misguided effort to show their concern for your baby. The truth is that you are responsible for your child, and the healthier you are, the better off your child is.

Bonding with your baby is important and fun, but so is self-care. Staying on top of my personal hygiene, health, and sleep (thanks to my husband, parents, and sister) made me feel cared for and confident. I think this supported my mental health, despite my history with depression.

Intrusive Thoughts

Trippy, creepy, and violent dreams and hallucinations are normal. Before I was pregnant, I had weird thoughts occasionally. After giving birth, I found myself having bizarre imaginings frequently. In my experience, it was not a reflection of how I felt about my baby or my husband. I was experiencing intrusive thoughts. This is normal especially for women in postpartum.

Intrusive thoughts are unwelcome involuntary thoughts, images, or unpleasant ideas that may become an obsession, are upsetting or distressing, and can feel difficult to manage or eliminate (Wikipedia).

Dr. Debra Kissen states that "Somewhere within an obsession is the flip side of a core value. If OCD taunts you with images and thoughts about offending God, then religion must be important to you. If OCD reviews all the ways your family could be hurt, then your family is clearly one of your top priorities."

I would confide in my father about the awful ideas I had. He never judged me. It was so helpful to tell someone I had terrible violent ideas. I didn't give him the graphic details, but it still improved my mindset. If there is someone in your life that you can trust not to judge you and to understand that it doesn't inherently make you a danger to your child, and to recommend professional support when necessary; I would advise you to confide in them. And, therapy can be very helpful.

PHYSICAL THERAPY

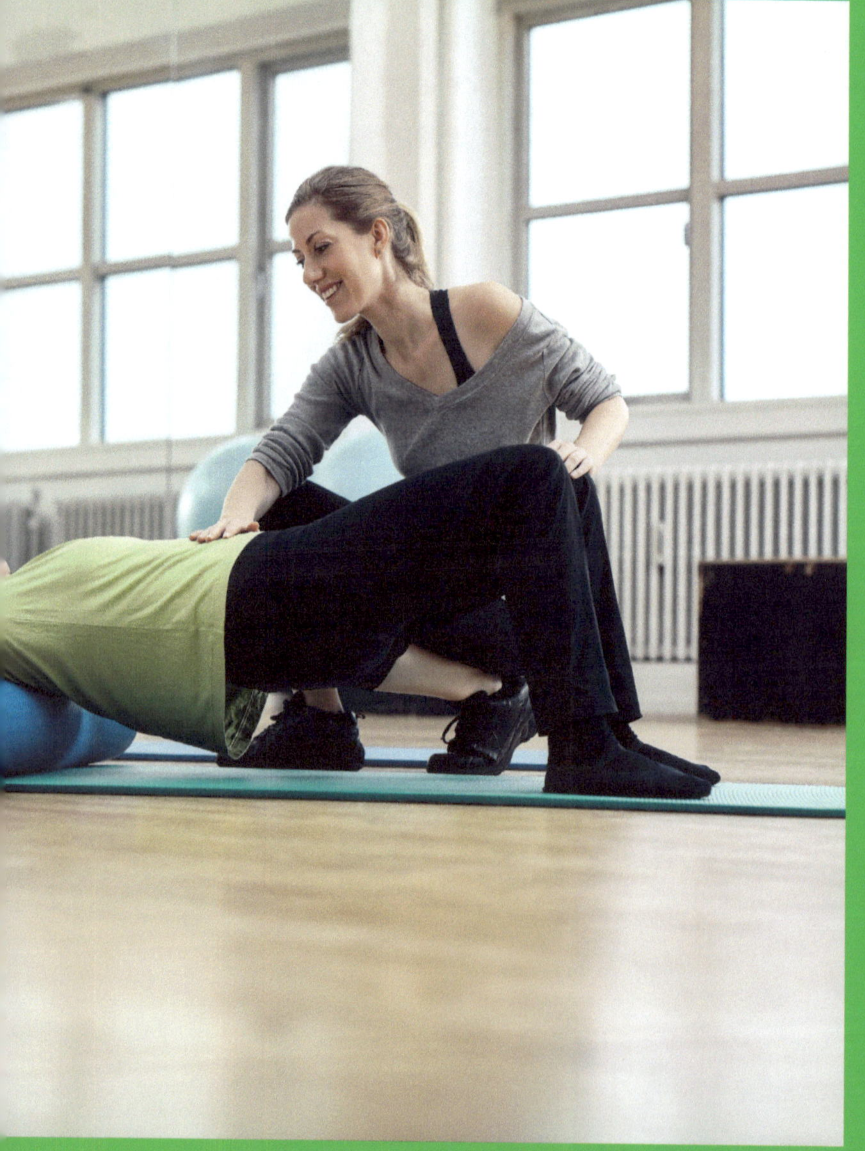

Physical Therapy

Despite what many people say about how long healing should take, I believe we all heal in our own time. Be patient with yourself.

Diaphragmatic Breathing

In order to restore your strength, and activate your transverse abdominal muscles, you should breathe deeply from your diaphragm. Many people tend to hold their breath when they lift something heavy or bend down. It may be necessary to pay attention to your breathing to make sure you are not holding your breath. It's healthy to exhale as you experience the most difficult parts of your movement.

Posture

It is important to have good posture to regain your strength. When standing and walking your feet should be parallel. Your knees should be loose, instead of locked. Also, don't tuck your butt.

Massage

Massage your vaginal lips with your fingers after your stitches have healed. Physical therapists recommend the use of the Laura Berman vibrator covered by a non-latex glove with organic lubrication internally to stimulate blood flow and promote vaginal healing.

Stretching

Doorway stretches, child's pose, legs up the wall pose, and supine twist help relax your muscles, and alleviate back and hip pain as you regain your posture. Foam rollers are excellent to keep your muscles loose, and relieve pain and soreness.

You can learn to do doorway stretches by watching this video: https://vimeo.com/231461660

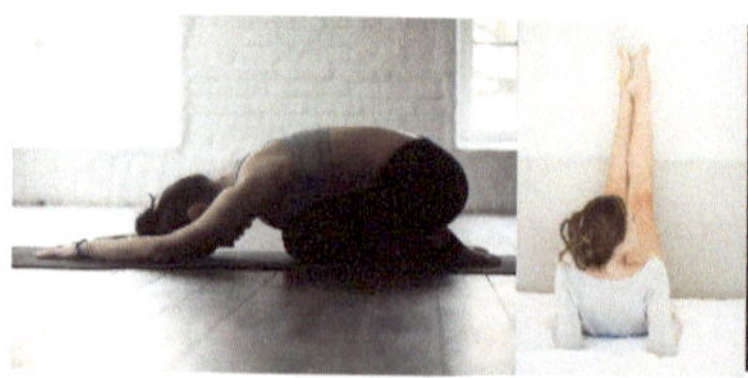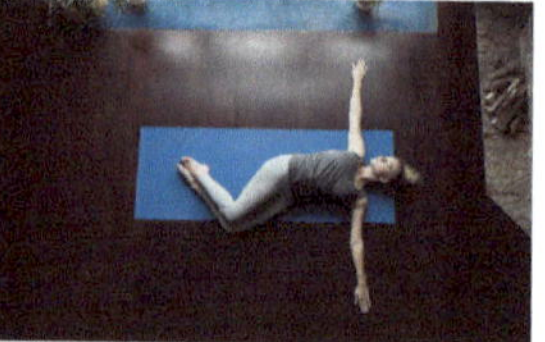

Kegels

Do kegel exercises by tightening your pelvic floor muscles for 3 to 5 seconds and releasing your pelvic floor muscles for 3 to 5 seconds. The pelvic floor muscles are the muscles you use to stop urination. It is important to strengthen your pelvic floor muscles because they support your uterus, bladder, small intestine and rectum. This is especially helpful if you experience bladder leaking after pregnancy.

Diastasis Recti

If your transverse abdominal muscles are separated more than a one finger width, you have diastasis recti. Your doctor can check for this at your follow up appointment after delivery. You can check it yourself by lying on your back with your knees raised, and placing two fingers just above your belly button while doing a slight crunch.

You may need surgery to close your diastasis recti if it does not resolve with time and exercise. I experienced diastasis recti. I went to physical therapy at an office in Illinois for help closing it. I got stronger, increased my balance, and relieved all my pain, but I wasn't able to close my diastasis recti until I began doing hook lying pelvic tilts.

Diastasis Recti Correction With Towel (Hook Lying) According to the Pelvic Health Rehabilitation Center's blog, "The patient takes a towel or bed sheet, wraps it around his or her waist, and crosses it at the largest gap in the DR. For most people the largest gap is at the belly button. The patient must hold the sheet nice and tight, making sure the sheet is in between the ribs and hip bones as they can hinder the sheet from being as tight as it needs to be. In that position, the patient does mini-sit ups.

Patients need to do 30-60 DAILY repetitions for the DR to close. The purpose of the sheet/towel is to bind the muscles together while the sit-ups strengthen the muscles in the correct position and close the gap. Doing sit-ups without a towel or sheet will cause the gap to widen."

After closing my diastasis recti, except the area around my belly button, I learned that I had an umbilical hernia that was repaired with robot-assisted laparoscopic surgery. We are all unique. Don't let your health journey discourage you. Try to find respectful health care practitioners you can trust. If you have limited options, use WebMD to do your own research and understand the health risks associated with your concerns. Also, fight to get adequate care, and ask practitioners to write notes in your chart that show that you have requested care. This is documentation to support that you are being denied care. Stand up for yourself. Don't settle for living with health risks that can be reasonably treated. That little drooling baby is counting on you. All my love.

Bonus Mommy Tips

1. To prevent your baby from falling, put him or her on the floor. They need tummy time for development anyway.
2. Treat baby scratches with Mederma to prevent scarring.
3. When your baby cries, ask yourself if the baby is hungry, dirty, tired, or lonely. If your baby is fed, clean, safe, and does not have a fever; comfort the baby patiently. Sometimes babies cry. Just consider each possibility and call your pediatrician with any concerns. My baby's doctor told me to take him to the hospital if he cried for an hour and was younger than three months old. Once he was older than three months, I was told to treat fevers and teething pain with baby Tylenol.

Shopping List

1. pads
2. witch hazel
3. aloe vera
4. lavender oil
5. Preparation H cream and wipes
6. Mederma
7. foam roller
8. belly band
9. sitz bath
10. sitz bath mixture
11. Desitin
12. rubbing alcohol

The End.

References

https://pelvicpainrehab.com/female-pelvic-pain/2306/fix-diastasis-recti/

https://www.healthline.com/health/womens-health/postpartum-belly#losing-belly-weight

https://adaa.org/learn-from-us/from-the-experts/blog-posts/consumer/how-take-power-back-intrusive-thought-ocd?page=1

https://proactivept.com/physical-therapy/blog-importance-hydration-physical-therapy

Credit
https://pixabay.com/vectors/pregnant-silhouette-lady-mother-3612889/
Mohammad Hassan

Stock photos provided by Canva.com.

www.ingramcontent.com/pod-product-compliance
Lightning Source LLC
Chambersburg PA
CBHW041805260726
48664CB00034B/427